Stop Feeding the Food Vampire

By

John and Lorraine Moran

Published by Stacked Deck Publishers

The book is dedicated to our son, John, for his support, understanding and help.

We also dedicate this book to every courageous man and woman that refuses to abandon their dreams.

Authors Note:

Consult a physician before beginning any exercise or diet program.

You are not alone. We suffered the self-doubt, anger, frustration and highs and lows you are experiencing as a Food Vampire and as the person desperately trying to cope with the obese individual. Sharing our raw and painful journey our hope is that you will regain a new strength and perspective and move ahead to a happy and healthy life.

This book is uniquely divided into two sections. The first segment is for the person struggling to maintain a healthy goal weight. The second section is for loved ones that face the daily heartbreaking challenges of dealing with the overeater plus easy healthy recipes and self-improvement log pages.

Table of content

Chapter 1

The addiction

All my life there have been more ups and downs than a playground swing. Each swing back to weight gain I deluded myself into believing I could handle the problem by saying, "I can stop overeating anytime." Unfortunately that stage of self-awareness was a long while in coming. First I had to get to know myself.

Everyone has three faces, one you show to friends another you show family and the other you show yourself. Getting to know myself was one of the most difficult undertakings of my life.

For years I maintained records of food intake and a daily journal of my trials and success. At that time the journal kept me on track, but soon I ignored the daily posts. Red flags of overeating were mounting on every page that became as commonplace as wiping away grease from the corner of my mouth. I stopped thinking about what I was writing. The journal was fed to the shredding machine while wishing I could turn back the clock.

As a teen aged boy I weighed 165 pounds earning a black belt in Karate. At the age of eighteen I was a Karate instructor and loved weight training. I leg pressed 1,010 pounds and lifted 605 pounds.

After a day of martial art training I ran home from the gym then ate anything I liked and didn't gain a pound of fat. Eating half a dozen hot dogs or hamburgers at one sitting was normal. Every day I drank protein shakes with bananas and globs of peanut butter added to the mix. At that time the phrase, "In Training," was a euphemism for Pigging Out.

This was my first lie. I had discipline in every other aspect of my life except food.

I loved food, but the affair soured. As I got older and consumed the same portions, food became a cruel mistress.

Let's explore the complex workings of the body to better understand the reasons we are hungry and why we don't lose weight.

It is called our bodies, "set point." The body gets accustomed to being heavier and when we lose weight it interprets it as starving. That is why starvation diets are the wrong approach.

Early man suffered seasons of famine and our body's conserved energy to sustain life. If the starvation situation continues the body begins to use the fat storage for energy. When the fat is no longer available the body begins to eat muscle to maintain life.

Look at photographs of World War II service men in prison camps, or victims of concentration camps. This is the result of the body attempting to maintain life by first eating the fat stores then cannibalizing the muscles. When the energy from these sources are no longer available the body dies.

Genetics may affect the amount of fat your body stores. Before supermarkets and readily available food, humans that could store more fat for the lean times had a better chance of survival.

When you go on a starvation diet the body doesn't recognize you want to lose the fat stores. Its primary directive is to stay alive. These diets are not only dangerous, but they don't work. You have to be on a healthy lifestyle of eating. Diet and deny are synonymous and that is why most people can't sustain them for a lifetime.

According to the Centers for Disease Control and Prevention, Americans are eating more calories per day than they consumed twenty years ago. It is an epidemic leading to hypertension, stroke and heart disease.

Using a Body Mass Index can determine obesity. It is an attempt to qualify the amount of tissue mass which is muscle, fat and bone that categorize it as underweight, healthy, overweight or obese.

Some methods to determine your Body Mass Index or BMI is through charts, skinfold thickness measurements with calipers, underwater weighing and bioelectrical impedance.

Your doctor should determine you ideal Body Mass Index.

Even if 2 people have the same BMI, their level of body fatness may differ. For example, at the same BMI women tend to have more body fat than men. Blacks have less body fat than do Whites and Asians have more body fat than do Whites. Older people, on average, tend to have more body fat than younger adults and at the same BMI, athletes have less body fat than do non-athletes.

Many factors are involved in weight loss or gain such as the environment, family history, genetics, metabolism, behavior and habits. While you can't change your genetics or family history you can change your lifestyle.

More than two hours of television viewing is linked to overweight and obesity. We rely on cars instead of walking, there are fewer physical demands at work and home because of modern technology and conveniences and lack of physical education.

Modern technology has made it easier to be inactive. Some of the things our parents and grandparents did on a daily basis burned calories and strengthened the heart, bones and muscles.

Cars didn't have power steering and automatic widows and mirrors. A push mower was used to cut grass and lawn trimming was done on the hands and knees using sharpened clippers. There were no snow or leaf blowers. Rakes and brooms cleaned the yard, steps and sidewalk.

To heat the home they shoveled coal into the furnace several times a day. Shopping and marketing was not done by pressing an app button. Everything was done physically and they interacted with store owners and cashiers.

The act of typing on a manual machine and pushing the carriage back took more energy. Each time our parents wanted to change a television channel they had to physically get out of a chair and walk across the room. There was no twenty-four hour programming, no endless sports stations so our parents and grandparents weren't staring at the television all day and night. Games were physical. You either went outside or you played board games which entailed interaction with people, reaching for game pieces, rolling dice as opposed to pressing buttons on a remote device.

They hung clothes outside which involved bending and reaching. No dishwasher. They stood by the sink and scrubbed and dried the china and silverware. Refrigerators had to be defrosted which meant empting the contents, allowing the ice to partially melt, then chop it away from the inside of the freezer. More meals were made from scratch as opposed to today's prepackaged foods filled with additives, chemicals, sugars and fats.

I'm not saying we should go back to the lifestyle of the past, but awareness of things you can do every day to be more active may help you not only reach your goal, but maintain a healthy weight.

Other factors are work schedules, oversized food portions, fast food in gas stations, movie theaters and supermarkets.

STOP FEEDING THE FOOD VAMPIRE

Portion sizes can trip you up. One half cup of mashed potatoes or the size of half a baseball has 112 calories. How many times have you piled a mountain on your plate and drowned it in gravy?

One ounce of potato chips is 152 calories. Even though the bag may say it contains three serving sizes, in reality it is one. How many times did you finish the entire bag without thinking about it?

One ounce of Swiss cheese the size of a pair of playing dice, not the kind hanging from the car mirror, is 107 calories. If you are like me, you crave cheese.

Today when I desire a cheese sandwich I buy the ultra-thin slices and limit the number to three pieces. My lifestyle has changed for the healthy and I'm not denying my cravings.

Let's explore this strange sensation called a craving. Cravings, hunger and satiety (feeling full) have a deeper cellular and hormonal origin.

It takes the body on the average twenty minutes to register it is full. Be mindful of what and how you are eating. Mindless consumption leads to overeating. Eat slower and chew food longer to help digestion. It will aid in the body's ability to tell you that you have eaten enough.

Leptin is a hormone made by fat cells. Leptin tells us to stop eating. Losing weight reduces Leptin.

Ghrelin is called the hunger hormone. These two hormones act in either opposition or teamwork.

The average person has approximately thirty billion fat cells. It is the largest army in the world and we are at war. As we lose weight the cells shrink, but don't vanish. Once we begin to eat more calories than our bodies can burn off, these cells again grow.

There are approximately one mile of blood vessels in a pound of fat. The number of blood vessels increases proportionately with the amount of fat we accumulate. Therefore, if you are fifty pounds overweight your heart must pump blood through and extra fifty miles of veins.

To lose one pound of fat we must burn 3,500 calories. Don't go into shock with this number. The calories can be burned over the course of a week by exercise and healthy eating. One to two and a half pounds per week is a healthy weight loss. In the beginning you may lose more weight and as your body uses the fat for energy it begins to conserve and loss may skip a week or only be half or a quarter pound. Don't be discouraged. Like it or not, this is nature's way of trying to protect us.

Sweet sugary foods spike the energy and then give you a quick low causing depression and the urge to eat more. Eating foods that make the body work harder to digest is another way of burning calories. High fiber

15

vegetables, fruit and whole grains will take longer to go into the blood stream and the body must burn more energy to digest the food.

Water plays an important part in weight loss and overall health. The body can only live a few days without water. Aside from helping fill the stomach, it lessens the burden on the kidneys and liver and dissolves minerals and carries nutrients throughout the body. Approximately 20% of our total water requirements come from food.

Some dangerous diets eliminate fluids causing dizziness, weakness, confusion, the inability to sweat, increased thirst and possible death. On average a man should drink about ten cups of water daily, a woman eight cups unless she is pregnant or breast feeding, then she requires more. You may need to drink more water if you are on a high fiber or protein diet, are in a hot climate or are losing fluids through physical activity.

Fat is essential to the body. Let's discuss the difference between saturated and unsaturated fat.

Saturated fat is typically solid at room temperature such as butter. Saturated fat raises LDL or bad cholesterol in the blood. Low levels of lipoprotein is associated with heart disease and stroke.

Unsaturated fat typically is liquid at room temperature but starts to turn solid when chilled. An example is olive oil. It is believed to lower the risk of developing heart disease and stroke. It also contains beneficial nutrients such as vitamin E which reduces bad cholesterol levels.

Our addiction is different from an alcoholic or a drug user. People addicted to alcohol or a drug don't require having a drink or the drug in the house, but a food addict must feed his addiction or die.

According to the New York Journal of Medicine gaining weight may be a socially contagious event. According to thirty years' worth of analyzed information, 12,000 volunteers were weighed every two to four years. The conclusion was that the risk of becoming obese rose nearly 60 percent for people with an obese friend and 40 percent for someone with an obese sibling and 37 percent with an obese spouse.

Well-meaning friends and family members have said, "Leave a little food on the plate. Use smaller plates. Drink water before the meal."

"You gained more weight." They made this statement expecting it to be a totally shocking revelation to me. Did they think I had no mirrors in the house? Did they think I had dozens of pants in increasing sizes because I was entertaining a troupe of circus clowns?

I also heard the monikers, "Fatso, tubby and big guy," and was assaulted with jokes.

STOP FEEDING THE FOOD VAMPIRE

1. When you went swimming did a bunch of whale watchers stop and take pictures?

2. You're so big you have your own zip code.

3. The only way to take your picture is on landscape setting.

4. I heard an elephant got loose and the keepers are coming to capture you.

5. You're so fat the bathroom scale cried.

6. You're so big you have your own gravitational field.

Why friends think it is O.K. to make jokes about your weight I will never understand. "After all we are friends and don't mean anything by it," they say. They expect us to laugh good naturedly at their wit, pigeon holing us into the stereotype that fat people are jolly people.

These statements make us feel miserable, hurt and wanting revenge. We are angry at those who hurt us and angry at ourselves.

Unfortunately, in dealing with feelings we too often eat to smother our emotions. After a lifetime of dealing with this issue I firmly believe the best revenge is success.

Here is where I want to pause and give you time to begin your journey to a better place. I have always been the type to bury my emotions, but discovered to get on track I had to face them.

Acknowledge and list the discomfort of rejection.

    1. Someone jokes about your weight. How does it make you feel?

Chapter 2

Humorless Declarations

For years the humiliation of the jokes had the opposite effect. It became a trigger to suffocate my emotions. Instead of swearing off binge eating and fatty foods I plunged in with a fork in each hand.

No one wants to be fat, hell I was obese tipping the scale at 310 pounds. How did this happen, how could I allow it to happen? I kept asking the question over and over then diving into the pity pool.

I married my high school sweetheart and we have a wonderful son. Both have supported and encouraged me, but none of that mattered when it came to my obsession with food.

I went to doctors, swallowed diet pills, went on crazy diets and joined recognized weight loss groups and organizations. The pounds came off, but after a few months I gained back more weight than when I originally started. The cycle of binge eating would begin again.

It is common for us Food Vampires to consume enormous amounts of food at one sitting such as a whole roasted chicken and stuffing, two dozen hamburgers, a jumbo jar of peanut butter, a bag of chocolate peanut butter candy or an entire brick of cheese even though we know it is a dangerous life threatening behavior.

When coworker's daughters sold Girl Scout cookies I purchased double the amount so I could eat a box that day and take the other home.

Ridding the house of red flag foods or treats can be one approach. Treats that I constantly craved that were at easy reach were too tempting. Lorraine stopped baking peanut butter cookies during the holidays and I stopped buying Girl Scout cookies at work.

1. **List the foods most likely to test your self-control and what you can do about them?**

2. List your weight gain justifications.

3. What was your method of dealing with the situation?

Chapter 3

Sneak eating

My wife, Lorraine, made good nutritious meals and I would eat my portions like a good boy, then sneak eat. When she was out of the house or in bed for the night I ate half a dozen slices of cheese filled with peanut butter wrapped in bologna.

Our dogs loved it when I had my sneak snacks because they licked the spoons and ate anything that dropped to the floor. They were my cohorts in crime cleaning up the evidence.

The prospect of discovery added a new twist to the insanity. My favorite sport was eating without getting caught while Lorraine was in the next room.

The dogs were a problem because they wanted the food so I devised ways of getting around that issue by saying I was getting treats for the dogs. All the while I was

27

wolfing down as much food as possible in the shortest amount of time.

Time was also part of the game. Sprinters time the distance from the start to the finish of the race and choking down food was my Olympic sport. More than once I was doubled over in pain, but kept eating faster before the pain became unbearable.

Food had a telepathic connection to my brain. It called to me from the refrigerator or the shelf and like a Vampire I craved the smell, taste and texture. No matter how I fought the urge to stay human and in control, the Vampire always won.

One holiday Lorraine made peanut butter cookies and I ate them all. At those moments for a food Vampire salads are a universe away.

She made a second batch of cookies and hid them in an attempt to stop me from eating them before guests arrived the following day. I waited until nightfall when she was sound asleep and like Dracula I crept onto her side of the bed, quietly slid the cookie tin out from under the bed and tip toed downstairs.

Sitting in the dark as the sweet pea-nutty goodness with green and red sugar sprinkles succumbed to my will I felt both good and bad about my cunning and success at purloining the treats. When the last cookie was eaten I thought about Lorraine. How was I going to explain this Vampire Food larceny? She was going to be angry, no doubt about it.

In the morning there was nothing to explain, the empty tin said it all. The only thing I could think to say in defense of my actions was a compliment meant to cast the blame away from me. "Lorraine it is all your fault for baking such delicious cookies. If you didn't want me to eat them you shouldn't have baked them." It's a foregone conclusion there's no need to describe her response.

29

A quick last minute visit to the supermarket and we had instant Christmas cookies for guests. No one seemed to notice or care they weren't Lorraine's homemade cookies and pointing out this fact didn't soften her mood. If faced with the same situation I would do the same thing and Lorraine knew it.

List the methods you use to feed your obsession.

Chapter 4

Routines are not so routine.

I created many yardsticks to compensate for my weight gain such as moving my belt out only one notch and vowing it was the last time. When there were no more notches I cut holes in the belt. I sliced seams in my socks to make them fit and loosened my pants to be more comfortable.

Soon bigger changes were needed. I wore a tie and a button down shirt. The tie was necessary to hide the shirt straining against the buttons. Before long I wore nothing but pull over tops to solve the problem the tie could no longer hide. Finally I had to buy bigger pants. In order to wear stretch pants comfortably I had to cut the waist. I started at size 36 and graduated to 46.

I had trouble reaching my feet to put on shoes so I bought a large spoon from the dollar store to use as a shoe horn. Later I wore only shoes with Velcro so they could be slipped on and off.

Clipping my toe nails was a major undertaking. Aside from the Kamasutra postures needed to reach my toes the procedure took forty minutes to complete. To get up and down stairs I needed a cane.

Another party favor of obesity was high blood pressure, one hundred eighty over one hundred ten to be exact. That still was not enough incentive to make a meaningful life change. I lied to myself believing I could enjoy binge eating for a few more days. Each time a makeshift solution to a problem was solved I always promised myself this was the last straw. Tomorrow I was going to eat healthy, exercise and shed the pounds.

Thinking back the situation reminded me of a story of two men sitting on a porch for hours until one finally moves and says, "That nail I was sitting on really hurt." The other man inquires, "Why didn't you move hours ago?" To which the second man replies, "Until now it didn't bother me enough."

Up to this point in my life the inconvenience, discomfort, loss of energy and health and the self-loathing was not bothering me enough to do something about it.

Those lucky people that don't have a weight problem see our lack of doing something about the weight as a mark of laziness and lack of willpower and courage. We put on an act it doesn't bother us, but it stabs at our core like a rusty knife. We do care, we have tried again and again to lose the weight. We are courageous in the fact we fail, eventually pick ourselves up and keep on trying.

My son said it best. "Food addiction is hardest to overcome. An alcoholic can stay away from bars, purge the house of wines and spirits, but food is always in the refrigerator and pantry."

Every other television commercial is about food, holiday celebrations are centered on food and a fast food joint is only a block away from wherever I travel.

After trying all the diet plans I am making it clear that I'm not supporting or trashing any particular group, organization or diet formulas. Some are good, some are bad and some are dangerous.

Before choosing a weight loss program do your research. Does the plan have flexible food choices, are the weight loss goals set by health professionals, are your food likes and dislikes considered in the plan, what is the percentage of people that completed the program, does the program offer support and counseling and finally are there additional fees or costs for items such as dietary foods and supplements?

I was very ingenious in creating food plans. One was extremely bad and I warn you not to try it. The idea was to eat less, but only the foods I liked. The brilliant plan was to eat one meal consisting of cookies, cakes, peanut butter or anything else I could think of for that meal. The rest of the day I would eat what my wife prepared.

To my surprise this diet plan didn't work. I soon realized a box of cookies for lunch or an entire large bag of potato chips didn't help me lose weight.

My quest finally took me on the path of studying food, but no matter how much I puzzled over the facts, joined support groups, the weight always came back with a vengeance. First the scale dial stopped at 208, then jumped to 232, onward and upward 256, 293, and 310. On more than one program I lost one hundred pounds, but it came back like a giant boomerang.

There is no question we lie to ourselves. We have all promised, "I'll start on Monday, the diet starts after the holiday, it is my birthday, I'll start tomorrow and today I deserve it."

Consider what you really deserve. Do you deserve the guilty feeling of failure? Is it a cookie or a piece of candy or do you deserve something better? If your answer is still the cookie, candy, pie or chips have the best. Don't skimp. Be satisfied. A simple fact is, treats that don't have salt, sugar, fat and other flavors taste like cardboard. This isn't going to satisfy you. Have your treat guilt free then go back onto a healthy eating program the rest of the week.

I finally hit rock bottom, but it wasn't just one thing that pounded the jack hammer of reality into me. For forty years I attended a local magic convention. My friends and I would stand outside and talk about the latest techniques in magic. For the first time in my life I had to sit on the building steps. I was in too much pain to stand.

When visiting my son in North Jersey he wanted to give us a tour of the town. It was a lovely sunny day and the view of the mountains was breathtaking. I deluded myself into thinking I could do it all. After walking one block I was out of breath and my joints were screaming. My son offered to walk home, get his car and take me back to the apartment. Pride wouldn't allow me to accept his well-intentioned offer. My irritability meter was high and I groused at my son and wife. It wasn't fair and neither deserved it. The truth of the matter is I was angry at myself, but unfortunately those closest to me bore the brunt of my self-loathing.

A half hour walk became a painful hour as I refused to turn back. We stopped at a restaurant for lunch and I soothed my bruised psyche with a hearty meal.

Einstein said, "Time is relative," and the walk back to the apartment seemed like it would never end.

The next day the plan was to visit Stevens State Forest. While Lorraine and John walked the nature paths I located a bench approximately fifty feet from the entrance and parked myself there and waited for them to return.

STOP FEEDING THE FOOD VAMPIRE

I was fed up and almost ready to change. Coming back from the trip we stopped at a restaurant and I ordered a cheese omelet, home fries, toast and scrapple (my local favorite delicacy).

That night while nursing throbbing joints I knew if I continued on this path I would die. There could be no more excuses and no more pity parties. I had to embrace that change comes slowly. It is a marathon not a race.

I told myself it can be done. The overwhelming number of pounds I had to shed wasn't going to stop me. I had to stop focusing on how long it would take to lose the weight. Even if it took two years to reach a healthy weight I had to consider what my life would be like in two years if I didn't take charge. I chose a Saturday afternoon to change my life around. Why afternoon? I'm so glad you asked.

I felt like a condemned man having his last meal. My farewell breakfast consisted of four eggs, mashed potatoes, hollandaise sauce and two and a half pounds of scrapple. It was such a pivotal moment I took a picture of the mountain of food.

What strategy did you use to deal with a

disappointment?

Chapter 5

Taking the first baby steps.

I didn't want to know how many pounds I had gained. I hate the charts and cringe when a nursing assistant announced my weight as I stepped off the scale.

The number would have overwhelmed me and led to depression that would have started me on another eating binge. Instead someone weighed me, but didn't tell me the result. My guess is it was two full spins of the scales dial.

This time I had to remember the pain both physical and emotional. No more lying to myself or playing the game, "this doesn't count," because everything counts.

Every day I wrote down each morsel of food consumed. Embracing the reason I wanted to be healthy had to remain first and foremost in my mind. It is so easy to forget why we want to be a normal size. I didn't say thin, I said normal.

One time I lost the prescribed weight a program stated was my goal, but I looked emaciated. The program didn't take muscle mass into consideration and as my wife pointed out muscle is more dense weight than fat.

The body works harder to supply energy to muscle than to fat. A person with more muscle mass burns calories more efficiently.

As a boy I was told not to put so much muscle weight on because once I stopped exercising it would turn to fat. That statement is totally false. Muscle cells will not magically transform into fat cells. Lack of exercise and poor eating habits adds fat cells and reduces muscle mass.

My wife was told weight lifting made a woman muscle bound. A woman will not be muscle bound unless she is taking male steroids. Estrogen keeps the female body defined. Weight bearing exercises will burn calories more efficiently, but she will not become grossly muscled.

The point is to choose a goal weight both your physician and you agree is healthy.

Your doctor may recommend keeping a food diary in which case you can choose the old pen and paper method or go digital. There are a number of free apps available, MyFitnessPal, LoseIt, MyNetDiary and MyPlate. Some allow you to scan bar codes on products to know the nutrients and calories consumed. While most apps haven't gone through rigorous scientific validation studies you should get a good approximation of your daily calories.

Like you, I still love to eat. At the writing of this book the problem is handled for now, but this is the part that scares me the most. In the past I kept the weight off for up to one year before tumbling off the wagon.

Now I immerse myself into learning new things to take the place of eating. I take on line courses in language, astronomy, Japanese culture and physics.

There are thousands of things to learn to challenge and excite you. Find the one that is right for you.

I created a set of life rules so I will never forget the steps of my journey. You may use mine, add your own or create a whole new list.

1. Don't Lie

Own up to the fact you are fat. If you pig out admit it. You're not a bad person.

2. Write It down

If you swallow it the amount matters. We fool ourselves by saying, "I'm just taking a little taste." Did you swallow it or spit it out after you tasted? If you swallowed, you ate it.

3. Recognize it will take forever

There is no such thing as, "I made it now I'm done." We have this problem for the rest of our lives. Once we stop we will gain it all back.

4. Have small goals.

Look at one minute, one day, one ounce at a time and it is more manageable. If I hadn't taken that approach I would have been defeated the moment I stepped across the starting line. Aside from the weight loss I was determined to be taken off blood pressure medication.

5. Don't expect miracles.

I weighed 310 pounds and lost ten, but realized no one noticed because it was like lancing a pimple on an elephant's rump. This was not going to discourage me. The hoopla and fanfare of others was not the purpose of this lifelong venture.

I was doing this for me alone. In the past I lost weight for my wife, my son, my job and it didn't last.

6.   Have a Daily goal.

At first it was enough to just get through the day. Later it was exercise. I walked half a block, a whole block and then two. Now I work out at the gym five times a week and walk four miles.

You may prefer other activities. Whatever you do keep it fresh and real. Getting into a rut is a guarantee you will stop exercising. At this very moment hundreds of pieces of in home gym equipment are gathering dust or substituting as a coat rack.

7.   Have fun.

Understand you are doing this for you and you are worth it. Make a game of your weight loss venture. Reward yourself. Buy something frivolous, take a trip, do something you have been putting off for another time.

8. Refuse to let failure define who you are.

Mistakes are a part of life. So what if you went off and ate until you felt like a tick about to burst. Move forward in confidence and put it on your shelf of life lessons. Yesterday has nothing to do with what you will eat today. Don't permit it to matter. Start again and practice self-compassion.

9. The perception of others.

People that don't have a weight problem feel that loosing should be enough of a reward, but sometimes it is not. There is the issue of depression because control isn't what we think it should be. We have mood swings.

10. Enjoy the little things.

One of the reasons I love my wife is the smallest things delight her. She enjoys the life that flourishes around her. It doesn't matter if it is a tree, dog, squirrel or lady bug. Lorraine sees beauty in everything. She taught me to enjoy a sunset and sitting in a park to watch ducks.

In the past my reward was mountains of greasy, fatty or creamy sweet food. I attempted to ignore the urge by eating a salad, a piece of fruit, but it didn't satisfy and soon I was raiding the refrigerator. I felt denied, angry and rebellious.

If food is going to be a reward it has to be something we really want and in moderation. A man once told me nothing smells or tastes better than cholesterol sizzling on a grill. If you want a steak don't cheap out, eat the best cut of meat. Don't skimp on a treat. Eat the brand of chocolate, potato chips or pastry you crave. Your reward should be totally satisfying.

While keeping my basic joy of gathering my wife, son and grandson close to me this new skill helped me appreciate life's wonders as well as lower my anxiety level. There was time to walk and laugh, time to kick off my shoes and feel the grass beneath my feet.

1.   Add your Life Rules to the list.

2. What makes you happy?

Chapter 6

Structure and discipline

In order to achieve my goals I needed structure and discipline. By nature I'm obsessed about time. If someone says they will call at 8 p.m. I am upset if they call at 8:01 p.m.

Sticking to a rigid regiment works for me. For example, I eat breakfast one hour after I awaken, 11o'clock sharp is lunch. My dinner is served between 2 and 4 p.m. after which time I work out at the gym. I allow for healthy and tasty snacks before bedtime.

I've listed a typical day's meal which you can try or create one that works for you. You may consider purchasing a scale to weigh food. A scale helped me not to underestimate or exceed portion sizes I calculated were essential to my goal.

Breakfast: A packet of instant hot oatmeal made with hot water or a rice cake or two eggs cooked in a spray butter substitute.

Lunch: Two pieces of reduced calorie bread with mustard, three pieces of ultra-thin cheese, four pieces of ultra-thin bologna and a salad minus dressing. You can use a low calorie dressing, but I don't like the taste or the extra calories.

Dinner: 6 to 8 ounces of beef, chicken, pork or fish and all the vegetables I want. I love hot sauce and use it in place of catsup, butter on baked potatoes and salad dressing.

Evening Snacks: Reduced calorie yogurt, red grapes or blueberries, blackberries, strawberries or a banana and two rice cakes or three pretzel sticks. Sometimes I indulge in two cups of popcorn in place of the rice cakes.

At one time I teased Lorraine. Her evening snack was a salad. To me an evening snack was a dozen jalapeno poppers. All that has changed. Lorraine remarked on the transformation because now I warm up the left over vegetables from dinner or eat a salad as the evening treat.

Once a week Lorraine and I go out for dinner or snacks and drinks. These are the days I spend extra time in the gym.

I plan for holidays and birthdays in advance by reducing the amount eaten for breakfast and lunch. For example, after enjoying everything I planned to eat and drink this past New Year's Eve, it was back to maintaining discipline and control. At one time I wouldn't have stopped until every last slice of pepperoni, cheese, crackers, and pie was eaten.

A weight range must feel comfortable. Discuss this with your doctor or a dietician.

In the past a few pounds of weight gain was ignored. More weight piled on and it was dismissed. Today I have set a range of five pounds. This is my red flag warning to immediately go back on my weight loss plan.

Within any given week the body experiences fluctuations of weight, some due to medications, water retention, sickness, lack of exercise or simply overeating. Not allowing the minor gain to snowball into an avalanche is my solution.

I work out at the gym four to five days a week, lift weights three times a week for approximately ninety minutes and participate in yoga classes twice a week. Even though I hate cardio I do my best to weekly walk four to six miles on the treadmill. After the workout I relax in the pool and hot tub.

My wife is a big believer in cardio cross training. An example of cross training is day one the treadmill, day two a low impact aerobics class, day three recumbent bike, day four swimming and day five the elliptical machine.

You should create a routine that works best for you. If you are like me, you simply can't use some of the machines. They aren't kind to my joints that suffer from job related injuries.

If you are new to a gym take advantage of the service of a personal trainer or trained staff member to explain the proper use of the equipment. What you don't know can hurt you.

Overdoing physical activity or engaging in strenuous exercise without properly preparing can lead to sore, stiff or pulled muscles, back injuries and heart attacks. It is recommended you speak with your family doctor before beginning your exercise and weight loss journey.

Lorraine worked in a gym for many years and was always amazed at the misinformation. She will not intervene when a man is trying to gain macho points with a lady unless the demonstration turns dangerous.

One man hadn't a clue what to do and was instructing the lady to sit backward on a machine which could have resulted in injury. Another man fancied himself a personal trainer minus the certificate or the training. He placed an elderly lady on a treadmill with a severe upward incline and a walking pace that would be equivalent to a marathon runner.

Here is where I feel compelled to speak about my gym pet peeve. Rest is important between lifting sets and depending on the routine it can be sixty seconds to five minutes in length. The issue irises when people hog a machine for a twenty minute gab fest. It defeats the guidelines of a proper work out as well as being ignorant of the needs of people that are serious about exercising.

Cell phones are an obsession. People talk during the work out, standing in the shower and sitting in the sauna. Recently I observed a man checking his phone text while urinating.

People, like it or not we are not that all important to warrant being connected 24-7. These individuals are oblivious of everyone and everything around them.

One lady so upset by something in the phone conversation made strangled sounds of anger and shock, planted her feet firmly and stopped moving. The treadmill did not.

Distracted members have dropped weights breaking bones in their feet or hitting people nearby. Preoccupied people in the gym are not only annoying, but are a danger to you.

Now all that is off my chest let's get down to what you can do to make the workout a more productive time.

Writing down the mileage walked and the calories burned is a great help as memory can fail you. Machines usually will give you a ball park idea and some programs will ask for your age and weight to be more accurate.

Over the counter heart rate monitors, activity and calorie counters may help to keep your exercise routine on track. They come in all price ranges and some are more accurate than others. Ask gym members that use these products what they recommend, check consumer testimonies and the Better Business Bureau.

Needing goals to keep exercise challenging and fun I create games. For example, can I beat the amount of repetitions or weight previously done on a particular machine? How much longer can I hold a yoga pose in the pool?

Rest is just as important to the body as exercise. When you lift weights muscle fiber is torn. A period of recuperation will rebuild the muscle tissue and it will be stronger. After a day or two away from the gym I always feel stronger and more energetic.

At the age of sixty eight I feel alive and happy. I came a long way from the man that could hardly walk a block.

We are masters at making excuses to avoid exercise. A classic justification is, "there is no time and I'm too busy." I said the same thing until I got it into my head that this is a marathon not a race. The key is to look to the future, not back to last week or last month. There is no free ride. We make the choices to change, have fun doing it and reach our goals.

You're not alone in the things you feel and nobody can tell you how you should feel.

When my goal to no longer need blood pressure medication was finally achieved my first impulse was to celebrate with food. Rather than the ravenous attack of a

Food Vampire, I took control by choosing what I ate, in what quantity and then regulated the meals for the week.

Keeping it real is one way I pick and choose what I will eat. Working off the calories of one slice of regular cheese requires walking on a treadmill at three miles per hour for twenty minutes. Calories consumed equals calories burned.

For years I wondered if green vegetables such as lettuce and Brussel sprouts are so good for the body, why they don't taste better. Give a child something sweet and creamy like ice cream they will want more. That same child offered a spoonful of Brussel sprouts will likely spit them out.

Finally, I have an answer to that question. An article in a men's fitness magazine stated our ancestors learned that sweet meat meant food was higher in calories and salty food would replenish electrolytes. The fact our ancestors didn't know an electrolyte or calorie from a rock didn't matter. They associated these foods with feeling healthy.

I must stress I don't cook because my wife will no longer allow me in the kitchen. Once I tried a recipe that called for corn starch. I put way too much into the pan then got distracted. When I returned the recipe was a solid burned block of something so inedible I could have used it as a door stop. The pan was ruined and the house smelled of smoke. Lorraine was not happy, but forgave me. Anybody can make a mistake.

After the corn starch fiasco I twice set the room on fire making popcorn. You can understand her wisdom in the matter of keeping the combination of me and the kitchen stove off limits.

I have let go the idea I can cook, eat anything anytime without structure, the games and the denial. I have let go the people that are detrimental to my happiness and success.

1. List the things that you can let go.

2. How does it make you feel?

3. Itemize your exercise routine for today.

4. Itemize a food plan for today.

Chapter 7

Perfection is a myth and accepting help.

It's time for a Reality Check. Is anything negative going to change your life? Would the world come crashing down if you failed? The answer is, only if it is permitted to live in your mind rent free.

How do you feel after losing five pounds? Do you expect to instantly look different to others? What do you feel when nobody notices? How do you deal with compliments after you have lost an appreciable amount of weight?

Each of us faces different challenges. One most people don't think about is the compliments and pats on the back as friends and family members begin to notice that you have shed a large number of pounds. We thrive on the attention and affirmation we did a good job. It was hard, time consuming and sometimes painful. With a flush of the cheeks and a humble, "thank you," response you soak in the adulation like a giant sponge.

Sometimes I wanted the praise to continue so I responded, "Wouldn't it be funny if I lost all this weight because I had a wasting away disease?" This joke was met with laughter and statements such as, "Only you would say something like that."

Comedy and tragedy go hand in hand so when I joke about myself I am alleviating the anxiety by controlling the situation. You laugh with me not at me.

What happens when people stop noticing? What do you do when the, "You look great," exclamations cease? Taking the weight off is the easy part compared to keeping it off. It is a life long journey and if you can only thrive on compliments you are in trouble.

Everyone wants recognition of the struggle and success, but is that the reason you are losing weight? No.

Adopt the mindset that people finally accept you as a person of a healthy weight.

I wondered about the people that never said an encouraging word or refused to notice my accomplishment. After deliberating the issue I discovered many were either jealous or were my biggest detractors. I was no longer an object to poke fun about to build up their self-esteem.

At the writing of this book I am struggling with both above mentioned issues. All the best meaning advice in the world won't help if it doesn't apply to your personal situation. You have to take stock in yourself and ask the question, "What am I going to do about it?"

You can enjoy yourself if you plan what you will eat and not go crazy. Plan and work your plan. So many people use the excuse they are too busy. Create your plan during television commercials, in place of texting or surfing the internet. Eating is one of the most intimate things we do that we have total control.

Another benefit of healthy eating is it helps memory retention. As long ago as 1983 adults ages sixty to ninety-four ate a wide range of nutritious foods and performed best on memory and thinking tests. According to the findings at the New Mexico School of Medicine, overall good food habits seemed more important than any one particular food or vitamin.

Letting go at times is important, just don't let go for the entire day. I have a friend who has kept one hundred pounds off for thirty years. He eats what he wants, but only one meal, usually dinner which consists of **one** serving of the desired protein and a desert.

Accept help

Abraham Lincoln said, "People are about as happy as they make up their minds to be."

It's not unusual to experience times of depression and it is a good idea to plan ahead for these moments.

Instead of wallowing in self-pity have an activity prearranged. Visit a park, play a game of chess, learn a language, take a course in painting, woodworking, golf, origami, learn to play an instrument, anything to avert your attention from your melancholy mood.

Approximately one in four people experience some form of depression. Natural chemicals effect your mood. Dopamine is a chemical that makes you feel alert and energized. Serotonin can make you feel calm.

Sometimes there is a malfunction in the body's ability to handle these neurotransmitters effectively. Sometimes we need professional help finding that happy place. Your doctor may prescribe antidepressants, MAO inhibiters or another medication to help balance your mood.

Exercise increases muscles, reduces the amount of fat stored in the body, and strengthens the bones and increases brainpower as well as being a good mood stabilizer.

Low impact and moderate activity will increase your heart rate and breathing. Participate in a water workout class, a chair aerobics class or a low impact group exercise class, walk briskly, bicycle on a level path or dance.

Many insurance plans offer free gym memberships. It is more cost effective for them to keep people healthy than to pay for medications, surgery and hospital stays. If your insurer offers this additional benefit take full advantage of it.

Friends and family members may offer well-meaning advice. They may suggest you join them in a project or activity. Instead of a defensive response try to understand and trust these people are trying to help you. They feel just as overwhelmed as you, but unless the project or activity is something pleasurable it is best to decline the offer and state the pastime you instead plan to pursue.

Avoid blaming yourself and others. It is a way to justify poor choices. Not everything can be cut and dried simple. What is best for me may not necessarily be ideal for you.

Your doctor may recommend surgery as a last resort to being overweight. Laparoscopic gastric binding surgery places a band around the upper part of the stomach creating a small pouch to hold food.

Gastric bypass surgery changes how your stomach and small intestines handle the food you eat. Not being able to eat as much as before the body won't absorb the calories so special care is needed to insure the proper consumption of nutrients essential to the overall body's health.

Liposuction is the surgical withdrawal of excess fat from local areas under the skin by means of a small incision and vacuum suctioning. While the fat cells are removed from a particular area without proper diet and exercise, cells in other areas of the body will increase in size.

If you and your doctor feel this is a good alternative there are excellent hospitals that specialize in these procedures. Usually there is a mental health professional available to answer your questions and concerns.

At one point I considered consulting my doctor about the procedure, but decided against surgery. After speaking to a number of people that underwent the procedure I realized it wasn't a magic bullet.

Some people gained the weight back after the surgery. If you want to cheat and overeat nothing can stop you.

1. **Identify the emotional changes you are experiencing of joy, confusion, depression, humor, conflicted and love.**

2. Write your exercise plan for today.

3. Itemize your food plan for today.

Chapter 8

Set Boundaries

Sometimes you just have to say "NO." Learn what things are important and let go of the rest.

We try to be everything to everybody and cannot fail at being a partner, housekeeper, breadwinner, spouse, parent, coworker, friend, confidant, and jack of all trades. Once we start down this slippery slope people expect it of us. Eventually we feel trapped, we don't want to let those depending on us down. The inability to escape causes depression and we turn to quick gratification which is food.

Trim away the unimportant, the things that you can let go or put on a shelf until a later date. Give yourself breathing room to collect thoughts, take stock and renew your energy. While most will be understanding, be prepared to weather disappointment, cajoling, or anger from people that don't understand or are too selfish to admit you are doing what is necessary for your health and wellbeing.

For me, announcing I was trying to lose weight was a big fat no. The declaration would have put undue pressure on me which could sabotage my efforts. Keeping my weight loss program close to the vest was an awkward business until I developed a few tricks I want to share.

When eating in a restaurant ask for low fat dressing or dressing on the side so you can portion out what you want. Ask for foods to be prepared dry instead of cooked in butter. Order baked fish instead of fried. Order a baked potato instead of French fries. Rather than butter, sour cream or catsup substitute hot sauces or mustard.

Saying, "I'm allergic" to foods that are on our stay away list is no lie. If you eat it you'll break out in fat. It has worked for me every time.

Sometimes people will try to pressure me to eat larger portions or consume foods I must avoid. After a meal my mother-in law always exclaimed, "Nobody ate anything. Look at all the left overs." Then she would ask me how much food I ate.

Following a weight loss program I knew exactly what portion sizes to consume, but it was never enough to satisfy my mother in law. I learned at family dinners as well as other banquets to politely state, "While it looks delicious I am full, but I may have something more a little later."

There is no need to go into lengthy explanations. Your reasons are your business. If they are true friends a simple, no thank you, should suffice.

In the not too distant past I orbited the tables always adding food to my plate. It was never enough. At one time my mind was in tunnel vision with the craving for that particular food paramount to the omission of everyone and everything around me.

When someone asks about your vacation and all you can recall is the food, this is a problem. Instead of speaking about the scenery, the culture or the historic landmarks you recount the restaurants and every meal in detail.

I still think about food. If I know a particular treat such as a pizza or a hoagie is on the menu I think about it. Today even though the Food Vampire is stirring I plan for the event and enjoy a moderate portion of treats and food. I don't deny my need to enjoy the banquet, but have replaced the obsession of thinking about food with enjoying the company of people around me.

Just because I have a plan doesn't mean the craving is gone. A magician didn't wave a wand and vanish all my road blocks.

What can you say no to today? List the things that are important and those that are not.

Chapter 9

Fear

We all have problems, money, jobs, children, relationships, and coworkers. Losing weight or being thin won't change these situations. Using these issues as excuses to overeat won't solve them, won't make them vanish into thin air. The end result will be the problem looming ahead of you and now you're depressed and fatter.

A little bit of fear is a good thing if properly managed such as the fear of gaining all the weight back again. I have learned to love who I am, but afraid of not improving who I am. My fear is the Food Vampire will return bringing with it complacency and being too satisfied.

I ask myself, "Is that what I want to return to?"

Before revealing one particular challenge I must first state that my wife has always been my number one supporter. I believe she doesn't have a mean or dishonest bone in her body. That being said, there were times I had fleeting thoughts she was insensitive.

I would be on my program and suddenly she was making corn bread, cookies and baked cheese macaroni. My first thought was, "Are you deliberately trying to make me fail?" When I verbalized the thought her response was, "It's not for you."

Not for me? All food was for me. Resentment was a good reason for me to eat. I thought she was doing this to test me.

Lorraine sometimes told me I had to wait to eat the forbidden food or I wouldn't get any. She was trying to teach me to take control, grow a pair. It had the opposite effect.

Now I realize she didn't want me to fail. This eating plan works for her and she failed to see why it wouldn't work for me.

Sometimes people will set up roadblocks to slip you up. On occasion friends tried to tempt me. They visited bearing my favorite trigger foods, something they never did when I was in pig out mode. They admitted it was a test. How dare they make a game of my life? Who do they think they are to quiz me? Finally I had to sever ties to these people to keep my sanity and live a healthy life.

You may have to take drastic measures to be healthy. Yes it is painful, feelings will be bruised, but you are worth it.

You must take charge and believe you are worthy of feeling happy and healthy. Support and weight loss groups can give insight, moral support and a yard stick to measure your progress, but it ultimately boils down to you. What are you willing to do for yourself? All the programs, diet charts, weigh in's or prepackaged meals will not be effective if you don't own up to your responsibility. You can't blame the world. You have to end the personal blame game and move ahead with life.

Life is goals and in our case small victories one day at a time. We will have occasional setbacks. They won't define us as failures, but mark us as courageous because we continue to work toward maintaining a healthy life. We can't let fear overwhelm us. We must make life changes to maintain our mental and physical health.

I'm grateful to my family because whether fat or thin they were always loving and caring. I always knew they would support me as I hope they know they are loved by me.

My final word to you is don't quit or feel useless. You have the power within you. You can stop feeding the Food Vampire.

Tips for reaching your potential

1. Get to know yourself both virtuous and flawed.

2. Try or learn something new or creative.

3. Instead of saying it can't be done figure out how it can.

4. Ask what is next. You can't sit back and expect everything to be roses and wine. The only constant in life is change.

1. **What self-help tip in this book helped you the most and why?**

2. What advice gave you the most trouble and why?

Chapter 10   Section 2

How it began.

My name is Lorraine and just like you, I wear many hats. I'm a wife, mother and grandmother, college professor of physical fitness, author and personal trainer. It has been a lifetime of learning, failures, success and introspect.

What qualifies me to know the issues troubling the overeater? How can I suggest coping methods living in an obese household? Life molds your choices. My past was a stepping stone to diving into physical fitness. I was an overweight child and my mother was overweight.

My grandmother struggled through the hardships of poverty and my parents grew up during the depression. Adults went without food so the children could eat a bowl of potato soup.

STOP FEEDING THE FOOD VAMPIRE

As a child I was surrounded by food, cakes, candy, cookies, and pies. I was encouraged to eat everything on my plate that started with a forkful of food named the train and my open mouth the tunnel. Then the peas, French fries, beans and noodles were personified into lonely creatures that would only be happy if they were eaten to join their family.

After dinner dad sometimes walked my sister and I to the ice cream store. Many Friday evenings he brought pizza home as an after dinner snack to eat while we watched our favorite television programs. It was an act of love that I took advantage of especially during the holidays.

My mom made the best apple pies in the world. She made tomato sauce and stored it in jars in the basement. Nowhere else in the world spaghetti and meatballs tasted the same. Every Easter the aroma of ham and baked cheese macaroni filled the air and Christmas tasted like her anisette pizzelle cookies.

I suffered the jokes and the emotions of one who doesn't fit in with the crowd and it wasn't just classmates that added to my unhappiness. Teachers, charm instructors and other callous adults added to the feeling I was trapped with no way out.

Suicide and the less permanent act of making myself deathly ill to alert people to my misery was considered. If not for a family that surrounded me with love I would have taken drastic measures to end the grief.

Raised in a household of devout Catholics I turned to God to end the unhappiness. I prayed each night that I wouldn't awaken. Alive the next morning I steeled myself for the misery the new day would bring.

Home was a sanctuary were I was accepted. Home was a place I never divulged my misery for two reasons. First I wanted it to be a safe place removed and unstained by the painful world past the front gate.

Second was the fear my parents would speak to the offenders and make life more miserable. Nothing is worse than kids thinking you had to run to mom and dad. It was risky allowing my tormentors to know how I was hurting. It would mean they won the fragile game between tormentors and tormented.

My mother offered to put me on a diet, but I refused. She was always on one diet or another. Nothing worked for her. Why should it work for me? There was nothing she could say that would make me agree to try to lose weight.

I was stubborn even though my heart was aching. It was a way to rebel, albeit the wrong way. Saying no gave me a weird sense of satisfaction. Nothing else in life was under my control.

I couldn't control the cruel laughter. My mother insisted on attiring me in dresses that had a sash and a bow that tied around the back. Those dresses made me look like

94

a gift wrapped beach ball. Each time I looked in the mirror

the rhyme, "fatty two by four can't get through the kitchen

door," played in my mind. What mom thought adorable

fashion was another nail in the coffin of my mental

wellbeing.

The more miserable things became on the outside,

the more food I ate. Feeble attempts to increase exercise

without curbing the calorie intake was a failure. Walking

or jogging a few blocks to the library didn't melt all the

pounds packed on from a hearty breakfast of pancakes,

butter, syrup and pork roll. Jumping rope for five minutes

or a dozen tummy crunches made no difference to my waist

line. Depression deepened and I lost all interest in the

things that once made me happy.

Sometimes I hugged my pound rescue dog, Lady,

and poured out my aching misery to her patient ear. She

was safe, my dog would never divulge secrets or tell me to

wipe away the tears and suck it up.

Finally I reached rock bottom.   My rock bottom was several things compiled into a potpourri of misery. The fattest boy in class told my how disgusting I looked. Until that moment I considered him a colleague in the outsiders club. The charm school teacher announced I was the most awkward girl in class. During the graduation runway walk fellow graduates undid the back of my dress. The thirty second walk of success became another joke.

My parents gave me the gift of a week on a horse farm. Finally I thought I found a sanctuary away from humiliation, but the owner and horse-riding instructor frequently made mention of my weight. I was separated from the other girls and forced to stay behind during night rides to clean stalls and brush down horses. It was embarrassing and I never told my parents. It had to be my fault that people were compelled to be cruel. I was convinced something about me was wrong and there was no place on earth to escape.

While shopping for summer dresses I got fed up wearing clothes from the chubby section. One last attempt had to be made to take control of my life. I held up three cute little summer shifts and promised my mother if she purchased the dresses, I would lose the weight to fit into them.

I can still see her sitting in the dressing room booth considering the proposal. Her eyes scanned the dresses and I held my breath awaiting the answer. She accepted my offer, purchased the dresses and that night put me on a reduced calorie diet.

It was difficult watching my sister eat ice cream while I chewed on a stick of gum. While other family members ate unlimited amounts of pizza, spaghetti, beef with tons of gravy, mashed potatoes, fried flounder, buttered macaroni, French fries, bacon, cheese, sausage, syrup and pancakes my portions were rationed. Whenever I felt my resolve weakening I looked in the closet at the pretty little dresses hanging next to the chubby girl fashions.

I exercised every day and each week my mother weighed me on the bathroom scale. By summer I fit into the dresses and liked my new body. It gave me confidence, grades improved and I felt renewed.

At school the boys persisted in getting close trying to get my attention and to find ways to sit next to me. The girls were jealous. I was the same girl, but with a different outer shell and no fool to the inner workings of the system. The classmates that found such joy at laughing at me had to find other victims to torment. Intervening on the part of their new prey and ending the bullies' fun became a mission I wholeheartedly enjoyed.

A few years later I gained all the weight back plus a few extra pounds. As a high school girl I decided to make a permanent change in my wellbeing. It was up to me to do something positive just for me.

I created an eating style that was livable. Exercise became an important part of the day. When I attended school dances held every Friday and Saturday night I was on the dance floor giving it my all. The pounds came off and I vowed never again to feel like a tick about to burst.

I have been on both sides of the road as an overeater and the daughter and wife of an overeater. I'm not bitter because it has given me a better understanding and empathy for people in both circumstances.

Maybe you have experienced similar situations or agonized over the same issues. Together we will face the emotions and search for solutions to the very real and sometimes overwhelming effects of living with an obese person.

Chapter 11

Setting down the rules to help the Food Vampire

I'll begin with the No list followed by positive things you can do for the Food Vampire. Later I'll give my life examples of how they worked and my mistakes.

The first thing to remember is always respect the overeater's food choices when they are on a healthy meal plan. Don't tempt them with a "bite" or a "nibble." Not only can this take them off track, but they could lose all control because at the end of the week, bites and nibbles add up.

Don't become the top sergeant of the food supply. You can ask them if they'd like you to help in this way, but don't be surprised or have hurt feelings if they refuse the offer.

Don't list out loud everything they eat or lock away or dispose of red flag foods you think they shouldn't have.

100

Humiliation and reprimanding them for eating the "wrong" thing is counterproductive.

Words can cut deeper and be more painful than a razor blade. While you may not be struggling with a weight problem yourself, consider the challenges the Food Vampire is trying to overcome. Think about how you'd feel if someone was always preaching and pointing out your flaws. Stop if these phrases are familiar. Did you stick to the diet plan today? You should have been more careful. Why did you eat that? What is wrong with you? What possessed you to eat like a pig? You blew it, happy now?

Don't attack the Food Vampire with weight loss books and articles, subscriptions to fitness magazines, or low-calorie cookbooks unless they ask for this help. Many well-meaning people overdo trying to be helpful. More is not always better.

Don't dwell on goals they haven't met. If they don't wish to talk about them don't bring them up.

Now that we have outlined the list of don'ts, let's consider the things we can do to aid the Food Vampire.

Encourage and cheer on the things they are doing correctly. An example is making mention of them reaching a goal or the effort of trying.

Eat some of the healthy foods with them, or at least taste the dishes. Good habits can become a normal part of every meal. Adding one nutritious food to every meal can be the first step to not only weight loss, but better health for the entire family.

If they join a gym or create an exercise program become an active participant in their healthy behaviors.

If they met a goal for the week or month, plan a celebratory activity that doesn't focus on food. Do something that reinforces spending time together, and create healthy activities that can further encourage their goals.

Let them know they can count on your caring and your participation in their life no matter what their size. Enforce the fact they can talk about anything that may upset them at any time and you will listen without judgement. Sometimes just listening and not speaking is what the overeater needs. Their speaking about issues diffuses the problem that would normally be smothered by food. Ask if they want your input, but be sure it is honest and constructive.

Chapter 12

Living with the Food Vampire

John and I met at the South Jersey Karate Club. At the age of sixteen I wasn't looking for a life partner, but after the first date I knew he was the man I would marry. He was kind, thoughtful, loving, athletic and strong and I felt safe in his company. Three years later we married and started a family.

The pressure of night school and working two jobs to support the family took its toll. Meal times were erratic and he started eating to calm down and reward his efforts. Meals were scoffed down to make deadlines.

At first the insidious changes weren't noticeable. He only gained a few pounds. On his days off we treated ourselves to the ice cream parlor for jumbo five scoop sundaes with all the trimmings or to a big breakfast at the diner.

The good wife that I believed myself to be had to reward my husband with food. This is what I was taught by example as a child.

On turkey day I made extra stuffing for John. I made additional burgers to stretch the food budget, but he ate them all at one sitting. He loved my baked macaroni and cheese and corn bread smothered in butter.

Peanut butter cookies are his favorite and one Christmas I made a double batch only to discover the next morning all were eaten. I couldn't bake cookies with him in the house because as each batch was taken from the oven, John ate them. After making the third double batch I was forced to put them in a tin and hide the cookies under my side of the bed to keep him from eating them overnight. He still managed to sneak them away and eat the entire contents of the tin.

At the time I didn't realize how serious the situation had become. John always had a hearty appetite and there was never a scrap of leftovers at the end of a meal.

He drove me to jazz dance classes because I am terrified of driving. While waiting for the class to end he visited the local sub shop and ate two American hoagies. After class I washed up and made dinner never knowing he had already eaten.

Soon he could no longer button a shirt or vest, larger size suit pants and jeans replaced the barely worn smaller sizes. John was out of breath going up the stairs. He had to stop and rest after walking one block.

Realizing this was a serious situation we spoke about an exercise program and healthy meal portions. I made salads, cooked with less salt, served more vegetables, less fatty meat, cut back on the purchase of cheese and peanut butter and we joined a gym for the summer. In theory that was a good start, but it didn't last.

I couldn't understand why he was still gaining weight. I didn't know he was sneaking snacks and hiding food. John was a master at manipulation treating the dogs to canine cookies as a cover to binge eating. I didn't know the few minutes delay in joining me in the bedroom at night, John was shoveling food into his mouth so rapidly he was doubled over in pain. Even when full he ate faster before the pain became unbearable.

Doubt about my sanity began to manifest. After finding an empty jar of peanut butter or cans and boxes of other items missing I began to question if I forgot to replace it on the shopping list. Maybe I did eat more peanut butter or cheese sandwiches during the week. John adamantly denied consuming the food, so it had to be a glitch in my memory. Why would he lie to me?

John was on the highest blood pressure medication dose the doctor could prescribe and still the readings were dangerously high. He was always out of breath. It was a real fear he would eat himself to death leaving me a widow. I went back to college to get a degree and took a refresher driving course should I find myself in an autonomous situation. At that point I believed I was racing against the clock.

Nothing I said or did made a difference. He stopped accompanying me to the gym and turned down offers to take walks. Instead of participating in moderate activity he napped in the chair with the television on.

On the days we went to a mall or supermarket John complained of hip joint pain. Rest stops became more frequent. He began leaning on a cane and considered renting a motorized chair to navigate the stores.

Several times he followed a weight loss program and there would be an improvement. At one point he was down to 170 pounds. I continued to prepare meals according to his diet plan and at first all was well. Then he would eat just one more piece of this or a larger portion of that. When we went out to eat and I couldn't finish my meal he began asking for a taste and then eventually consuming the rest so it wouldn't go to waste. When I questioned the behavior John said he knew how to handle it and not to worry. But I did worry.

He always marveled that I could eat and not be compelled to finish everything at once. We discussed the issue of an overeater and likened it to an alcoholic finding it remarkable a person could stop at one drink or have a bottle of whisky, beer or wine in the cabinet for months.

A good example is the Valentine Day he bought chocolate covered gourmet strawberries. I ate two large berries a night until they were gone. A box of candy or cookies lasts for months. It may take up to two weeks to finish a pie and six months to eat a box of ice cream bars.

As an overweight person in my youth, this plan of action worked. The treat is there and I can have it all or I can choose to spread out the enjoyment for days or months.

To my surprise, after having a particular treat available I no longer craved it. The mystic lure was gone.

Some stores such as those selling candy, chocolate or ice cream allow new employees to eat as much as they want. The forbidden treat is readily available and the overwhelming desire to consume it is eliminated. The companies understand denying the treat would only serve to increase the craving that would then become an obsession.

Chapter 13

Self-Preservation

It can be hard and heartbreaking to watch a family member or friend speeding to self-destruct mode. How to handle the situation can create stress not only for you but, for the person you desperately want to help.

You tried gentle prodding and it didn't help. The anger approach was as satisfying as a spit filled balloon dropped onto your head. Nagging, crying and threats made the situation worse and may have made the person so defensive they rebelled with a cheese steak and a double loaded order of cheesy fries and deep fried jalapeno pepper poppers.

The actions, failures, and success of the overeater shouldn't reflect on you. Eating is a personal experience and it is solely in their domain to abuse or control it.

It's normal, but not healthy to carry guilt and feel you have failed the obese person. You question if there is something else you hadn't tried, something you shouldn't have said or done.

The fact is, there is nothing you can do to force an over eater to adopt a healthy lifestyle. The effort will eventually take its toll on your body through headaches, tension, abdominal discomfort, and lack of sleep and reduced cognitive ability. Constant long term tension may shorten your life and can damage your heart. It affects sleep rhythms and impedes the body's restorative ability. Anger so intense you can't put your emotions into words is another way to sabotage your wellbeing.

Too often we neglect our needs to sacrifice for others, but it doesn't work for long. The outcome is that we suffer by putting ourselves at risk, damaging our health and relationships.

It is time to go into a self-preservation approach to deal with your emotions. Learn how to relax by defining what tension is in your body.

Are your jaws clenched, shoulders tight, is your breathing shallow and quick? When you climb out of bed are you still tired? Are you making more mistakes and are more forgetful? Do you have more frequent or severe headaches? Is the tension causing you to either over eat or have a loss of appetite?

According to a study at Tufts University, women are more prone to gain weight due to depression than men. Some believe it is because women may more readily use food as a coping method.

Focus on things you can do. Don't give up the enjoyment of life. It isn't selfish to make time for yourself. Even a computer needs time to debug and reboot. You will find you feel so much better both mentally and physically after quality me time.

For me, quality relaxing time is taking a walk, puttering in the garden, watching classic comedy shows, writing a novel, riding my stationary bike wearing headphones and listening to my favorite kick ass aerobic tunes or meditating to soft music with a scented candle flickering on the table.

People ask me how I felt when John got upset during his weight loss journey. As with most parties that disagree, each feels they are correct and the other person doesn't understand.

We rarely argue which is good because I am the quick fuse and he the slow burn. My major flaw is rocket and fire verbal outbursts. I do try to curb them and one way to dull my sharp tongue is physically putting distance between me and the individual targeted for the cutting words. Taking a walk gives time to gather my thoughts.

One occasion that stands out in my mind is a day out of the blue John asked to take a walk with me. After explaining the route and distance my walk usually takes he insisted on going.

With him in tow I was limited to a couple of blocks. The pace was leisurelier than I was accustomed and came to a halt numerous times so he could rest. John repeatedly asked me to walk slower. My hurtful response was, "If I went any slower I would be standing still." I was impatient.

Soon John declared he wanted to turn back for home. My walk had barely begun and I didn't want to head back so soon so I offered John the house keys.

Instead of going home he trudged on at a snail's pace in considerable pain. Should I have agreed to go home with him then headed out again? Should John have taken the keys and allowed me to finish the walk alone?

At the time I was angry and felt he was in the wrong. Why didn't he go back without me? Why did he have to spoil my outing because today of all days he decided to take a walk? Come hell or high water I was going to finish my trek even though the joy had gone sour. It was a cut my nose off to spite my face reaction.

John believed I was wrong for not accompanying him back home. At the time I didn't understand he was unsure if he could make it back. With this information I would have either offered to get the car or stayed by his side until he was back in the Livingroom lounge chair.

Although quarrels are rare, my feelings are always bruised. After a while I realize it took two to create the situation and a discussion follows. Sometimes I'm more in the wrong and apologize. Sometime John has to be more forthcoming about what he is thinking and feeling.

It is O.K. to sometimes feel angry. It's O.K. to sometimes feel a little selfish. What you do next is important. Do you allow problems, arguments or an uncommunicative person to color your entire day in shades

of grey or do you move forward?

1. Be in command of your feelings by putting them into words.

Develop an emotional vocabulary and use specific words to label your various feelings. Be honest with yourself as you create your list.

2. Let go of things that annoy you.

List the things that trigger your tension.

3. **What is your response to the things that annoy you?**

4. What are the ways you discovered to relax?

Chapter 14

Your Brain can lie to you.

First let's discuss the positive way the brain can tell lies. Using color when preparing and serving food helps to brighten the meal and create a healthier menu. The eye perceives the color as more inviting. For example when serving a white meat such as pork or poultry add orange, green or red vegetables to the plate.

The palate can be fooled by gradually reducing salt and fat or using salt and butter substitutes. Combining foods gradually can also help. Try blending cooked spaghetti squash to your pasta dish or puréed cauliflower to mashed potatoes.

Serving bland colored foods such as mashed potatoes or pasta on a colored plate as opposed to white will make the portion size more visible. It fools the eye and may help reduce the amount of food added to the plate.

122

The brain can be fooled in many ways. During a case study in Canada two groups of people were given a chocolate bar with a fruit filling. The first group was told it was a new health bar, the second was told it was a new delicious candy bar.

The group that believed they were eating a health bar claimed to experience greater hunger, while the group that believed they were eating a decadent calorie filled chocolate bar felt satiated or full.

Negative lies are imposed by the overeater. They believe they can quit overeating any time they want. Sometimes they underestimate the amount of food they consume and overestimate the amount of physical activity they have done.

It is not unusual for a person with an overeating problem to consume a box of donuts and convince themselves the two block walk home will be enough to shed the extra glazed calories. No amount of facts in books or on charts will make a difference. It is part of the

pathology. They lie to themselves. They lie to you.

As an ACE (American Council on Exercise)

personal trainer and college graduate of Exercise Science

it's not unusual to have clients sign up a month before

bathing suit season expecting to shed a years' worth of

weight gain. Some clients expect to follow a diet and

exercise program for one month and have the physique of a

dedicated gym member who worked for years to achieve

the desired weight and shape.

I never lie to them. If facts and explanations don't

work I indulged the service of a gym member the client

wished to emulate, requesting they reveal the number of

hours and months it took to achieve their goal.

I refuse to train them if they aren't willing to put in

the effort and work to achieve their goals. To agree to train

them under any other condition I believe is wrong. It would

be deluding them into thinking they can reach from the

basement to the attic in one step with the end result of depression and failure.

It is a rewarding experience years later to meet people that followed my dietary and exercise programs. To hear that I made a positive difference in their lives is gratifying.

Over the years I have spoken with many people that have a weight problem and to the people that worry about and love them. Some admitted they raid the garbage cans after family members have gone to bed, hide snacks around the house so they can eat undiscovered in the basement, attic or back yard shed. I discovered it is not uncommon to stand in front of the refrigerator with the door open eating everything on the shelves.

Giving away or trashing the red flag foods of the overeater was an exercise in futility. It sparked arguments, added to the tension and discord in the household and in the end the overeater repurchased the foods and snacks and ate more. The decision has to be one they choose to make.

Those that love the overeater told me of the tears, worry and feelings of helplessness that plague their lives. Some found support groups through the church, outreach communities or internet organizations.

Check the internet for support sites for the compulsive overeater and recovery groups for family and friends of the overeater. In the last chapter of the book we have included a number of sites that may be helpful in finding nutritional, weight and mental health help and information about associations in your area.

Chapter 15

Pitfalls and Pit stops

Unintentionally or consciously the road to a healthy weight can be sabotaged by family or friends. Sometimes our friends came calling bearing John's favorite forbidden treats well knowing he was on a diet. My intervention did little to stop the behavior. It only ended when John spoke up either ending the friendship or refusing to allow them to visit bearing these danger foods.

It was boring preparing the same meals and I decided to break out and make something I liked. Those treats were also John's triggers. My intention was not to upset his program or destroy his resolve. I really believed only making a small portion for me would do no harm. I also believed if I allowed him to have a small amount of the forbidden food it would satisfy and teach him portion control.

At that time he was in a very vulnerable state and to John it appeared I was acting cruel and insensitive. He accused me of sabotaging his diet.

Again my feelings were bruised. I began to doubt my intentions. Was I subconsciously trying to topple the tower of his determination to lose weight?

The lifestyle worked for me why not for John? The answer is my way isn't the only way. One size doesn't fit all. I had to allow John to get there on his own. Once I stepped away from the situation I understood my actions were counterproductive.

Realizing I had to be more sensitive to his disorder didn't mean following his diet. We had to agree upon a plan that would satisfy both of us.

Admittedly, I believed I should be able to do it all, always questioning if there was more or a better way to do something to help my husband return to a healthy weight.

In most cases I was upset at what was not accomplished instead of sitting back and saying it was a job well done.

The guilt cycle was driving me crazy. I hadn't learned to step back and come to grips my husband had to make the difficult decisions for his sake alone. He couldn't do it for me, our son or anyone else. I didn't yet understand it was more effective to wait for him to ask for help or advice.

Every suggestion was ineffectual. I appealed to a future where he wouldn't be here to see his grandson married, the possible heart attack or stroke before he knew the joy of holding a great grandchild in his arms. Not even scare tactics of a bed ridden life unable to walk to the bathroom or bathe was taken seriously.

There were breakthrough moments when he said he would try. He sought out support groups and on occasion created a diet plan in hopes that trial and error would produce a magic formula. He tried to analyze where he was succeeding and failing. After following a particular long but healthy program John lost one hundred pounds only to be plagued with the terror it would all end. He had learned how to lose the weight, but not how to live the life of a healthy person.

I praised his effort and encouraged him, but when he did slide back into his old habits my coaching and praise had the opposite effect. Trying harder didn't heal my husband's food addiction, shield him from the pain and cruelty of fat jokes, or show him the negative impact his behavior had on the family. With each failure I fooled myself into another round of mental sparring to find the solution.

To this day the fear of sliding back to his unhealthy ways is like a faceless specter of failure waiting in the shadows. Unlike my aversion and anxiety of driving, going back to his old ways is a real health issue.

We are human and will continue to make mistakes. We have ridden the guilt train and have been the guest of honor at more than one pity party. We've made ourselves miserable and questioned our self-worth. Past screw ups come back to haunt us like hungry living entities that we feed by the fistful.

As we lay in bed they invade our thoughts. For hours we stare at the ceiling as dozens of, "what if I had only" scenarios, or "why I didn't" plots jump into our brain like monkeys on a trampoline. It is counterproductive and at times I too still wrestle with them, but recognize there are options.

John and I have discussed in length that complex time and the pitfalls and for today have jumped the hurdle. I say for today because tomorrow will be a new set of challenges.

A good example is the challenge that winter weather poses. We tend not to go out as much on cold and snowy days. In the spring and summer John and I are more active outdoors whereas when days are short and roads are icy we become more homebound. The time for temptation to satisfy appetites increases. We try to overcome this craving time with activities other than watching television. Sometimes it doesn't work as well as hoped. Then we go into plan B which is waiting another hour and if the urge to eat a particular food is still there, a small portion and no more is eaten.

John realizes he has to face the addiction and at the same time enjoys the benefits of a healthy life. Today he is no longer in need of blood pressure medications.

He requested I bake peanut butter cookies for the holidays. The big difference is his attitude toward the treats. While the craving to eat the entire tin of cookies exists, John decided he would eat only three cookies per week and had me save twenty four in a plastic bag. The rest I gave away.

There will be many dinner invitations, parties and events and John has to stay focused and be responsible for what he consumes. He has to manage and choose regardless of what everyone else is eating.

In the end I realized the gold standard of effectiveness was being there when he needed love, understanding and support. Doing what he needed at the time and no more worked better than pushing for results.

John asks me to make homemade vegetable soups, salads, and bake fish and low fat meat. When I make spaghetti and meatballs he controls the amount of sauce and pasta on his plate or I prepare separate fresh tomato, mushroom and pepper sauce.

He has preplanned healthy filling snacks in the evening which includes a portion of fruit, rice cakes and fat free yogurts in various flavors to ward off boredom.

I occasionally make baked cheese macaroni and home fried potatoes. It is his choice to control a small portion or avoid eating these foods. To be fair I inform John of the menu in advance for him to plan.

Every day is a new challenge, a new set of surprises and upsets. It is what you do about them that is important. A very wise man once said to always ask, "What's next?"

See mistakes and failures as opportunities. Mistakes should not define you. Stop beating yourself up for failing. Consider how you would speak to a friend in this situation and apply it to yourself.

1. **List your mistakes and failures as if a friend or loved one was confessing to you. Answer them in a compassionate and constructive way.**

2.   **What is next?** List the things you can do to make

positive changes.

Chapter 16

Just the facts

It is important for you to keep healthy both physically and mentally, but how can this be done? It may help to understand the role the body plays in weight gain and the difference between hunger and appetite.

Hunger is the body's response to needing fuel to continue staying active and healthy. Appetite is the desire to eat regardless if hunger is present.

Other factors are at work such as Ghrelin and Leptin. Ghrelin also known as Lenomorelin is produced by cells in the gastrointestinal tract. Besides regulating appetite it plays a significant role in regulating and distribution of the use of energy. When the stomach is empty Ghrelin is secreted. When the stomach is stretched secretions stops. It also plays an important role in regulating reward perception.

Leptin or Attos Leptos is the Greek meaning for thin. Leptin is the satiety hormone and has the opposite effect of Ghrelin. It is made by adipose cells (fat) that help regulate energy balance by inhibiting hunger.

Both Leptin and Ghrelin act on receptors of the hypothalamus in the brain to regulate appetite to achieve energy. In obesity, a decreased sensitivity to Leptin occurs resulting in an inability to detect satiety or the ability to feel full despite high energy stores.

The average person has approximately thirty billion fat cells. As we lose weight the cells shrink, but they don't vanish. Once we begin to eat more calories than our bodies can burn off, these cells again grow.

There are approximately one mile of blood vessels in a pound of fat. The number of blood vessels increases proportionately with the amount of fat we accumulate. Therefore, if you are fifty pounds overweight your heart must pump blood through an extra fifty miles of veins.

To lose one pound of fat we must burn 3,500 calories. Don't go into shock with this number. The calories can be burned over the course of a week by exercise and healthy eating. One to two and a half pounds per week is a healthy weight loss.

In the beginning the obese person may lose more weight. As the body uses the fat for energy it begins to conserve and loss may skip a week or a couple of weeks or the loss may only be half or a quarter pound. Many times they get discouraged, but like it or not, this is nature's way of trying to protect us.

It may help you to understand the other reasons an overeater may not lose weight or as much as they hoped. The result is falling into discouragement, anger and despair.

An underactive thyroid or hypothyroidism slows down the metabolism. Cushing's syndrome is a condition in which the adrenal glands make too much of the steroid hormone Cortisol. In the healthy body Cortisol is released in response to stress, functions to increase blood sugar, and aids in the metabolism of fat, protein and carbohydrates.

Medications can cause the body to hold water and slow the rate the body burns calories.

Many people eat more when they are bored, angry, stressed and have stopped smoking. People that quit smoking claim food tastes better. Nicotine raises the rate the body burns calories and with the termination of the drug, the body's response is to slow the metabolism.

With age we lose muscle tone and muscle loss can slow down the rate the body burns calories. Midlife weight gain in woman is mainly due to menopause and lifestyle.

Not enough regular sleep causes weight gain. Hormones that are released during sleep help control appetite and the body's use of energy. For example, insulin controls the rise and fall of blood sugar during sleep.

People who don't get enough sleep have insulin and blood sugar levels similar to people with diabetes.

Before starting any weight loss or exercise program it is recommended the person consult their family physician. Simple tests will determine if there is a medical reason weight loss may be impeded and in most cases medications can be prescribed. Consulting a licensed Dietician may also aid in understanding proper portion sizes and menu planning.

There is sometimes confusion about the difference between simple, complex carbohydrates and dietary fiber.

Simple carbohydrates raise the blood sugar faster and higher. After consuming a simple carbohydrate the energy level spikes then quickly falls. The body then craves more to enhance energy. It is a vicious cycle. Simple carbohydrates are found in fructose processed food sweetener such as table sugar, candy, syrup and soda. Healthy foods such as carrots, potatoes and white bread have more simple carbohydrates than apples, lentils, peanuts and whole wheat bread.

Complex Carbohydrates found in milk, beans, beets, rice and fruit prevent binge eating and encourage weight loss because they are rich in fiber. It remains in the stomach longer, slows down and promotes digestion and keeps you satiated (feeling full) longer.

High fiber is a term used to distinguish the fiber in food from natural sources. These foods help to decrease appetite and may help lower blood sugar and prevent colon cancer.

A woman needs 25 grams of fiber per day and a man should consume 35-40 grams.

Some foods high in fiber are prunes, pears, apples, mangos blackberries, navy beans, black beans, pinto beans, kidney beans and canned baked beans, rye and wheat bread, bran flakes, almonds, walnuts and peanuts.

Add chopped walnuts or almonds to salads or sprinkle them in vegetable dishes. Replace sugar coated cereal with Shredded wheat and oat meal.

For dinner try a cup of whole wheat spaghetti, wild rice, or barley. Vegetables such as broccoli, winter squash, Brussel sprouts, spinach, sweet corn and peas can be stir fried or added to soups and stews.

This isn't a complete list of all the high fiber foods available. You don't have to be a head chef to create new and flavorful ways to prepare these foods. The internet, library and book stores are a great source of healthy meal planning with many recipes to choose.

Besides fiber the body requires nutrient rich protein. Men should have 56 grams daily, a woman 46 grams, teen girls 46 grams and teen boys 52 grams. Some people mistakenly believe more is better and either take protein supplements or overeat the recommended amount of daily protein required by the body. What the body cannot use for energy is expelled in urine. There is no benefit in the overconsumption of protein.

Three ounces of lean turkey, chicken or beef which is the size of a deck of cards is the desired portion size. Omega 3 which is a good fatty acid is found in salmon. Other protein sources are low fat dairy such as cheese, milk, and yogurt. Eggs and soy are an excellent source as are nuts, seeds, beans, peas and lentils.

Three ounces of skinless chicken breast has 25 grams of protein. Two tablespoons of natural style peanut butter is 6-8 grams. One cup of low fat cottage cheese is 10-14 grams. So you see, it isn't difficult to meet your daily protein requirements.

According to a study by Tufts University we must also consume folate. Folate is a water soluble B vitamin found in food. Since it is water soluble, it leaves the body through urination. Low levels of folate are thought to cause depression. Good sources of folate include green leafy vegetables and fruit such as strawberries and melons. It is found it dried beans, cereals, fruit juice and multivitamins.

It is believed obese persons are more likely to develop a folate deficiency due to the fact they do not eat healthy which in turn increases depression and the vicious cycle goes around and around.

While a multivitamin is recommended if you aren't consuming the required minerals and vitamins from food, you may consider a diet supplement. A word of warning about diet supplements is they should only be consumed under the supervision of a doctor due to the side effects from medication and overdose.

Many people don't like to drink water, but water plays a significant role in keeping alive and staying healthy. Water moistens the tissues in the eyes, nose and mouth, it lubricates the joints, regulates body temperature, flushes waste, lessens the burden on the kidneys and liver and dissolves minerals and carries nutrients through the body.

The body can last for weeks without food, but only days without water. The body is 50 to 75 percent water. The water content in men is higher and falls in both sexes as we age. About 20% of our total water requirements are consumed from food.

The daily fluid intake for men is ten cups, woman eight cups, boys seven to eight cups and girls six cups. You need a higher intake of water if you are on a high fiber or high protein diet, pregnant, breast feeding, physically active or exposed to warm or hot conditions.

Inadequate fluid intake risks kidney stones, urinary tract infections, and lower physical and mental performance.

Some of the warning signs of dehydration are dizziness, weakness, confusion, an inability to sweat, increased thirst and the urine is dark amber. Untreated death may occur.

Protecting your wellbeing and health takes planning, but it isn't rocket science. This is a partial list of some of the healthy low fat foods you may consider stocking.

Fat free or low-fat milk, yogurt, cheese, and cottage cheese, light or diet margarine, eggs or egg substitutes. Sandwich breads, bagels, pita bread, English muffins, soft corn tortillas, low fat flour tortillas, low fat, low sodium crackers, plain cereal, dry or cooked, rice and pasta.

White meat chicken or turkey (remove skin), fish and shellfish (not battered), Beef: round, sirloin, chuck arm, loin and extra lean ground beef, Pork: leg, shoulder, and tenderloin.

Dry beans and peas, fresh, frozen, canned fruits in light syrup or juice. Fresh, frozen, or no salt added canned vegetables. Low fat or nonfat salad dressings. Mustard and catsup, jam, jelly, or honey. Herbs, spices and salsa.

There is a marketing hype that has been very successful for many years. You have seen packages with bold print announcing the product is either sugar free, salt free or fat free. Many times the product never contained sugar, salt or fat. A good example is a bottle of water stated it was fat free.

Remember whatever is taken away from a product something else is added to enhance flavor. It is important to read the labels to keep yourself and loved ones healthy.

The newest marketing ploy is labeled Gluten free. According to the University of Chicago only three million people are affected by Celiac disease. But, considering the millions of people that do not have this autoimmune disorder or a wheat allergy there is no reason to purchase a Gluten free product. It is a case of marketing genius. They inundate our world with these commercials knowing a large portion of the food shopping adults will fall prey to the ads.

Shop smart and have your list in hand. The products the store wants you to buy are usually at eye level with colorful packaging. Other ploys to make you buy are placing non-essential items near the checkout counters.

Use your list and stay with it. Be sure to eat something before food shopping. Hunger will weaken your resolve making unhealthy or normally unwelcome food choices to end up in your grocery cart.

Chapter 17

To help you kick start a healthy menu I am sharing my favorite recipes that are fiber, protein and complex carbohydrate rich.

My crock pot vegetable soup recipe.

1 cup of fresh or frozen spinach or escarole

1 large red pepper

2 jalapeno peppers

1 cup fresh or frozen broccoli

2 tomatoes

1 cup fresh or frozen cauliflower

½ cup of peas fresh or frozen

1 15 ½ ounce can of pumpkin (Not pie filling) is optional.

Salt or salt substitute to taste.

For a more seasonal holiday flavor add ½ teaspoon of

cinnamon and nutmeg

Chop the vegetables into eatable size and place into a crock

pot half filled with water. Add the pumpkin. Season to

taste. Serve when vegetables are soft.

Tomato sauce substitute.

1 can 14.5 oz. stewed tomatoes.

5 to 10 sun dried tomatoes

1 cup chopped fresh mushrooms

1 green pepper

2 jalapeno peppers

1 onion

Fresh or powdered garlic to your liking

1 teaspoon Basel

1 teaspoon Oregano

Salt or salt substitute to taste

Olive oil

Pour 1 tablespoon of olive oil into a wok or pan set on medium heat and add chopped vegetables. Combine Basel, Oregano, salt or salt substitute and garlic.

Stir as mixture begins to bubble. To thicken add a ½ teaspoon of corn starch. Serve over whole grain pasta or spaghetti squash when sauce has a creamy consistency.

Adding two 10.5 oz. cans of drained clams, crab meat or mussels to the ingredients adds a flavorful change of pace to the dish.

My mom's Simple Summer Salad

3 cut tomatoes

1 sliced onion

1 teaspoon Basil

1 teaspoon Oregano

¼ cup of olive oil

Salt or salt substitute to taste

Place all ingredients into a bowl and put into the
refrigerator overnight to allow the flavors to blend. Mix
and serve.

Crock Pot Pasta and Beans

1 can baked beans drained

1 can black beans drained

1 can tomato soup add 1 cup of water.

1 chopped onion

Garlic (optional)

1 cup uncooked whole wheat elbow pasta

Salt or salt substitute to taste

Put everything into the crock pot on low to medium setting until pasta is soft and enjoy a healthy and economical meal.

For a heartier meal add tofu or 1 pound of ground beef, pork, turkey or chicken. Brown the meat in a pan with ½ teaspoon of olive oil, drain and place into the crock pot.

Mom's beef stew

1 lb. beef cubes

2 potatoes boiled until slightly soft

1/2 cup peas

4 tablespoons barley

2 stalks of celery

2 carrots

Brown beef cubes in ½ tsp of olive oil. Chop carrots, celery and potatoes into bite size pieces.

Add water to a pot or crock pot set on low heat and combine vegetables, meat and barley. Stir stove stew pot occasionally to prevent burning and add water as needed for the desired consistency.

Salt or salt substitutes are best added at the end of the cooking cycle as potatoes will absorb the salt if placed into the stew too early.

Meat loaf, meat balls, hamburgers and chicken.

Substitute oat meal for bread crumbs to add fiber and nutrition to your protein dish. For added flavor, fiber and moisture dice a fresh apple and mix it into the ground meat before cooking.

Use ground corn meal is place of commercially prepared bread crumbs when coating baked chicken.

Holiday Party Dip

1 pineapple

1 large container of non-flavored yogurt.

2 tablespoons of Shredded coconut (optional)

Scoop out the pineapple and place the fruit aside. Mix the coconut into the yogurt and place inside the pineapple.

Cover the pineapple and let mixture chill overnight to absorb the sweetness of the pineapple. As guests arrive place pineapple pieces, fresh sliced apples, melon and strawberries around the pineapple for dipping.

Chapter 18

No Mulligans / Set Boundaries

No doubt many of the experiences we shared in this book are upsetting and may have poked a finger into a very raw emotional wound.

It is important to understand while you can't force an obese person to make a life change you are able to take command of your emotions and health.

"Not my circus. Not my monkey." While it sounds simplistic the message rings true. The job of the obese person is to be the ring leader and we must accept the role of spectator even if the act unfolding is unpleasant to watch.

The stark truth is not every story has a happy ending. Unfortunately some will not live to reach rock bottom. For many loved ones this painful scenario has played out to the final conclusion. Obesity is at epidemic proportions and for this reason hospitals and mortuaries have super-sized scales, beds and coffins.

There are different rock bottom set points. It is the moment of epiphany when they choose life. It may be an impending surgery, wanting to fit into a dress or suit, deciding being chair or bed bound has to end or the desire to once again play a sport.

Sometimes you just have to say NO. Learn what things are important and let go of the rest.

Growing up I always felt like a bug under a microscope. My mother told me if I didn't dress a certain way, hang the clothes on the line a particular way or trim the lawn just so, the neighbors would speak ill of me. For some reason what neighbors and strangers thought was of utmost importance.

In all fairness, my mother had her demons. She always thought her apple pies were a disaster even though they were delicious. Even if you ate like a starving refuge she always believed you should eat more, there was too much left over to refrigerate. Not finishing everything she served was an aspersion on her culinary ability.

She was on every diet imaginable that ended in failure. She and my aunt had friendly competitions and as long as my aunt stayed the course, so did mom. She had to compete then revel if she lost more weight that week than my aunt. Once my aunt quit the diet so did mom.

Mom bought a crazy devise that shook and jiggled the fat around as you leaned against a thick belt. It didn't melt away the pounds as she hoped and later became a weird looking shelf for sewing material and patterns.

At that time dance and water aerobics classes were unheard of. Gyms were still considered a smelly sweat house where men pumped iron.

One day it dawned on me I had to let go of all the rituals. Mom's hobgoblins morphing into my life couldn't live rent free in my head. There was no vacancy for the manipulation and drama of childhood routines or the problems of current situations.

I don't have to be perfect or define self-worth by a dress size. If a task doesn't get done today it will keep until tomorrow or next week. Nobody outside my skin cares.

You may have worried what others think about you. The raw truth is most people don't give you a second thought. They are all wrapped up in their lives and no doubt a good portion of them are concerned about what you perceive of them. Any doubt or emotion you feel, everyone else is also experiencing. Wrapping your mind around that idea helps remove much of the separateness we experience.

We are not to blame or responsible for another person's actions. Life is too short to play the pity game.

Learn to say no to stressors and yes to joy. Feel energized

and take an interest in life's wonders.

Reach your potential.

    1. Get to know yourself both virtuous and flawed.

    List your insights

2. **Instead of saying it can't be done figure out how it can. What is your break through result?**

3. What issues have bothered you?

4. What self-help tip helped you the most and why?

Chapter 19

Helpful Sources

National Alliance for Mental Illness

www.nami.org

USDA Food and Nutrition information Center

www.nal.usda.gov/fnic

U.S. Food and Drug Administration

www.fda.gov

American Dietetic Association

www.eatright.org

The American Heart Association

www.americanheart.org

American Cancer Society

www.cancer.org

International Food Information Council

www.ific.org

www.ingramcontent.com/pod-product-compliance
Lightning Source LLC
Chambersburg PA
CBHW062207280526
45788CB00001B/477